Finding Personal Peace
Twenty-Eight Yoga Classes
For A Balanced Life

Finding Personal Peace
Twenty-Eight Yoga Classes
For A Balanced Life

Melissa J. Chaney

Printed in the United States of America

Library of Congress catalogues the title of this as follows:

Chaney, Melissa J., M.S., R.Y.T.
Twenty-eight Yoga Classes for a Balanced Life
        p.   cm.
        ISBN: 1469990652
        ISBN: 9781469990651
        1. Self-help – Yoga. 2. Yoga – Hatha Yoga- Ayurveda   I. Title

Publisher: CreateSpace
        Charleston, South Carolina
        www.createspace.com

DEDICATION

I offer this book to all my teachers throughout my life, especially my daughter, Ione, my son, Fynn. I also offer this book as a symbol of gratitude to all my students whom have taught me all about the human Spirit.

ACKNOWLEDGMENTS

I ACKNOWLEDGE: Patricia Hansen, Hansa, Dr. Lad, Chitra, Bethelya, and all practicing health educators and yoga therapists for their direction and support. Patricia, this book is your work in action, based on classes you have taught. You are my very first teacher in the arts and sciences of Yoga and Ayurveda. Through your wisdom, I learned to dance, the dance of life, love, and light. Hansa, I am indebted to you for influencing my concepts of Yoga. Thank you both for your acts of selfless service.

I ACKNOWLEDGE: You, the reader. In many spiritual communities, sangha, offers the opportunity for inner growth through the practice of spiritual lifestyle and spiritual practices. Therefore, one of the key elements is to surround yourself with others who are on the path for mutual support and learning. May you conscientiously develop spiritual aspects of your life.

CONTENTS

INTRODUCTION

The following suggestions are suitable for morning, late afternoon, and/or early evening yoga practices. Take time to connect to your inner harmony through the breath. Remember that breath always precedes movement. Be consistent in your practice and with perservance and humility and you will be rewarded. Every action is either a call for love or an act of love.

After 28 days, step out from this new sense of sacred space that you have created and see how you feel. Then pull back into that sacred space and stay there for a while. Keep your sacred space shielded and again work on what is right for you.

Yoga is a deliverance from pain and sorrow. When the mind, intellect, and self are under control and free from restless desire, one is in communion. Regular practice of your own sadhana and the presence of God follows. Make way for abundance, release yourself from fear, and open yourself to receive pure love.

When one has self love, one can have compassion for circumstances and can make decisions based on one's circumstances. Everything that is going on around oneself is their circumstance. There is a healthy way to respond.

We are in an ever-changing environment if we cannot change the external, we can change the internal. We always have the capacity to love, and "I" can choose to live in that love. When someone has self-love, you can meet people where they are with pure awareness and without judgement. Our yoga practice gives us a space to get out of our emotional responses.

I was taught to activate spiritual wisdom through withdrawing my senses inward. Allowing the mind to follow the path of breath which is where the lotus of the heart resides. Though your point of reference may be different, it is important to follow the procedure, yet the technique must be flexible. Your own inner feeling is your teacher.

Learning to properly sit, focus the mind, and the experiential process will enfold. When you travel through your heart, you will enter into the seat of transformation. This is the beginning of gathering energy into every cell which is the miracle of yoga.

Enjoy your inner exploration of body, mind, and Spirit! These twenty-eight practices offer centering prayers, asana, pranayama, meditations, and songs. May we all house the Light of the Spirit. Life may not be the party we hoped for ... but while we are here, we might as well dance!

Opening Prayers
From Satchidananda
Ashram-Yogaville

OM OM OM

Omkaaram Bindu Samyuktam
Nityam Dhyaayanti Yoginaha
Kaamadam Mokshadam Chaiva
Omkaaraaya Namo Namaha

Om united with the Source,
on which the Yogis ever dwell
Grants desires and liberations,
Salutations to the Omkaaram.

Gurur Brahmaa Gurur Vishnu
Gurur Devo Maheswaraha
Gurur Sakshaat Param Brahma
Tasmai Sree Gurave Namaha

The Guru creates. The Guru preserves.
The Guru dissolves the Universe.
The Guru, in fact, is the Absolute.
Salutations to the Sadguru.

Om Namah Sivaaya Gurave
Satchidaananda Moortaye
Nishprapanjaaya Saantaaya
Niraalambaaya Tejase

The Guru is Auspiciousness,
Embodiment of Truth- Knowledge – Bliss.
Salutations of Him who is beyond the worlds,
Peaceful, Independent, and Radiant.

Hari Om

Class 1
New Beginnings

- Opening Prayers
- Pigeon breathe in two breaths
- Standing warm-ups. Neck rolls on the right side in full circles and then to the center before making full circles on the left side.
- Lying on belly on the floor; experiment with the Feldenkrais technique. Outer arm at a forty-five degree angle, other arm is bent and head rests on arm. Lift head and arm together. Do several repetitions on each side. Come to the center and see how far you can look up. In this exercise imagine making complete figure eights with the spine.
- Sitting in hero pose, virasana, make figure 8's with the jaw. Massage almond/coconut for pitta and sesame for vata/kapha. Relieves TMJ, stress and whiplash.
- Lion pose, simhasana 3-4 times, removes wrinkles from face, removes fear.
- Forward bend, uttanasana
- Runner's stretch with arms to the inside, elbows to the floor.
- Downward dog, adho mukha svanasana
- Plank, caturanga dandasana
- Warrior I, virabhadrasana I, on knees arms behind ears
- Extreme forward leg stretches, utthita parsvottanasana
- Two arm, one leg balance, vasisthanasa, into pigeon, eka pada rajakapotanasana
- Deep Lunge
- Garland, malasana
- Intense leg stretch, prasarita padottanasana
- Wind relieving pose, pavanamuktasana
- Bridge, setu bandhasana, supported on all sides on the skinny side of the block.
- Stomach twisting pose, jathara parivartanasana
- Splits, hanumanasana
- Savasana, gentle Yoga Nidra
- Song, "Aidi Shakti, Aidi Shakti, Shakti Shakti Shakti, Aidi Shakti, Danuvad" "Thank You Great Mother"
- Closing prayers from Satchidananda Ashram-Yogaville:
- Lokaah Samastaah Sukhino Bhavantu!
- May the entire Universe be filled with Peace and Joy, Love and Light. May the Light of Truth overcome all darkness!

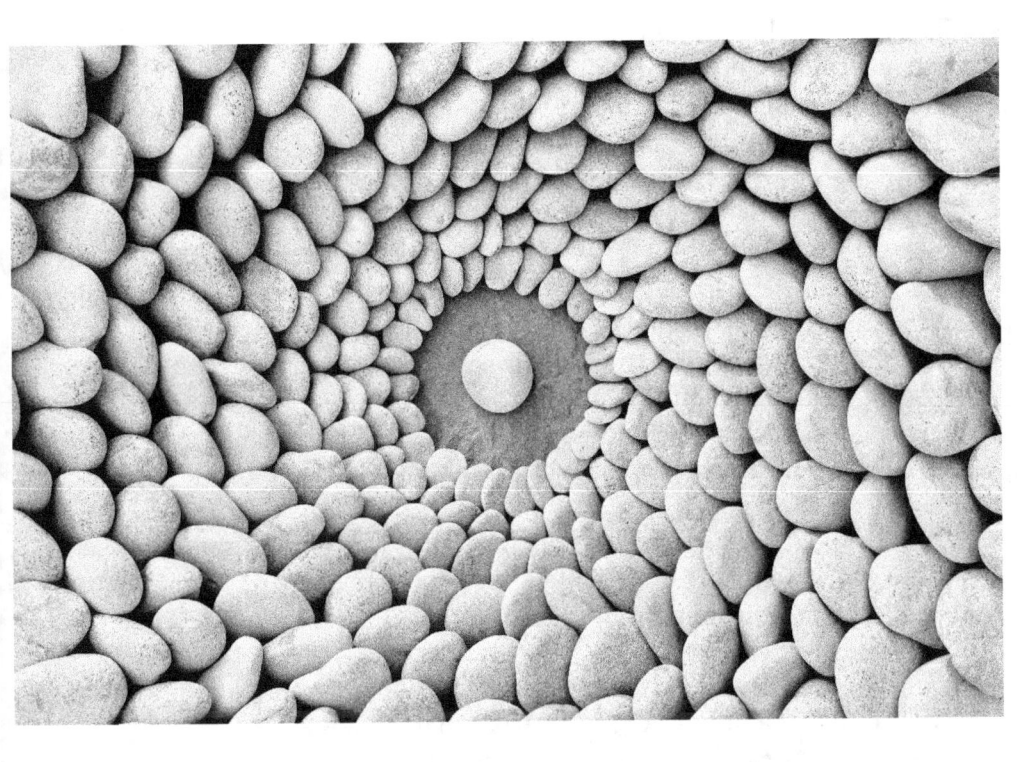

Class 2
Restorative Practice

- Opening prayers
- Standing Neck Rolls, five in each direction, lift chest
- Ashwini mudra, draw air out and hold
- Agni Sardoti, pump stomach
- Breath of Arjuna
- Shanti Mudra, Meditation on the Heart
- Affirmations in Temple breathing---
- "I am" ,"I am one" and, "I am one with the Universe."
- Chair poses with variations, utkatasana
- Mountain pose, tadasana step back into warrior II, virabadadrasana II
- Draw arms out behind back body into warrior I, virabadadrasana I (Both Sides)
- Legs 3ft. apart extended forward bend, padottanasana, clasp arms behind back and squeeze shoulders together.
- With the help of partner, rotate their shoulders out to open chest, pull arms up gently for extension.
- Bridge poses with a block, setu bandhasana. For depression relief, focus on the chest with emphasis on squeezing shoulders toward block. Try different block sizes.
- Vishnu, lying on the couch. Both legs and hips drawn in to stabilize back.
- Hare Pose, sasangasana into child's pose, balasana
- Boat, navasana on stomach, thumbs interlaced. This variation protects the back.
- Drop hands to floor, palms down, engage pelvis, legs and then lift arms, hands face one another. Another variation of boat pose.
- Locust, salabhasana. Thighs on floor, knees bent, arms rotate back and lift.
- Pelvis rocking on stomach in all four directions.
- Partner supported shoulder stand, salamba sarvangasana. Hold them by the ankles and roll them in and out of supported shoulder stand.
- Savasana
- Yoga Nidra
- "So, Ham" Mantra Meditation 10-15 minutes
- "Danyavad, Danyavad, Danyavad, Ananda," "Thank you for awareness of bliss."
- Closing prayers

Class 3
Serenading the Divine

- Opening prayers
- Standing, Breath of Arjuna
- Affirmations in inverted Namaste' Mudra, Temple breathing
- Shanti Mudra, Temple Breathing with affirmations, "I am one," "I am one with the Universe," "I am the Universe." At root, at heart, at crown.
- Aura clearing
- Forward bend with hands under feet, padahastasana
- Toe Balance; roll on tippy toes and balance.
- Runner stretches into sun salutations, surya namaskar
- Warrior II, virabhadrasana II with bow and arrow. This posture strengthens thymus gland.
- Hands/Arms 14 inches forward on floor, lift one leg at a time into half moon, ardha chandrasana
- Standing half moon, ardha chandrasana
- Boat, navasana, working with the breath lift legs and then arms
- King cobra, bhujangasana with knees bent, feet together
- Frog stretches; mandukasana; lying on stomach reaches back and grab one foot and stretch over hamstring, both sides.
- Dolphin, catur svanasana
- Downward dog with arms on the floor, adho mukta svanasana
- Frog, mandukasana
- Child's pose, balasana
- Pigeon variations, eka pada rajakapotasana
- One hand to foot
- One elbow to foot, followed by two arms to one foot
- Both sides
- Pelvis rocking while seated imagine the belly of bowl of cherries, roll in all 4 directions.
- Seated boat, navasana, with shining skull breath, kapalabhati
- Kapalabhati breath seated in sukhasana
- Savasana
- English Folk Song...
- "I love you whether you know it or not,
- I love you whether I show it or not,
- There are so many things I want to share inside my heart,
- And now is a great place to start."
- Closing prayers

Class 4
The Bhagavad Gita & History of Yoga

- Opening prayers
- The Bhagavad Gita, *The Song of the Lord*, inserted between chapters 25 and 42 of the great Indian Epic, The Mahabharata.
- The History of Yoga
- The Vedas- oldest Scriptures of India 2500-600BCE
- 4 Vedas, each has four parts
- Shat Darshan- Six insights into the nature of reality: Yoga being the fourth
- The 5 Kleshas: Yoga Sutras-Mirrors to freedom
- Yoga postures for total health:
- Cobra, classical, bhujangasana
- Cobra, arms folded behind body, fingers interlaced, bhujangasana
- Locust, shalabhasana
- Boat, navasana
- Bow, dhanurasana
- Child's pose, balasana
- Downward dog, adho mukta svanasana
- Child's pose, balasana...rabbit, sasagasana...child's pose, balasana
- Hero, virasana ... seated forward fold, pascimottanasana
- Symbol of Yoga, yoga mudra, seated in a comfortable position
- Son of the Creator pose, marichyasana
- Savasana
- Meditation, "Golden Globe above Head"
- Sufi Song....
- "I rejoice in your Light Lord, as the Moon reflects in the Light of the Sun. Oh, La, Oh, Oh, La, Oh, La, and Oh."
- Closing prayers

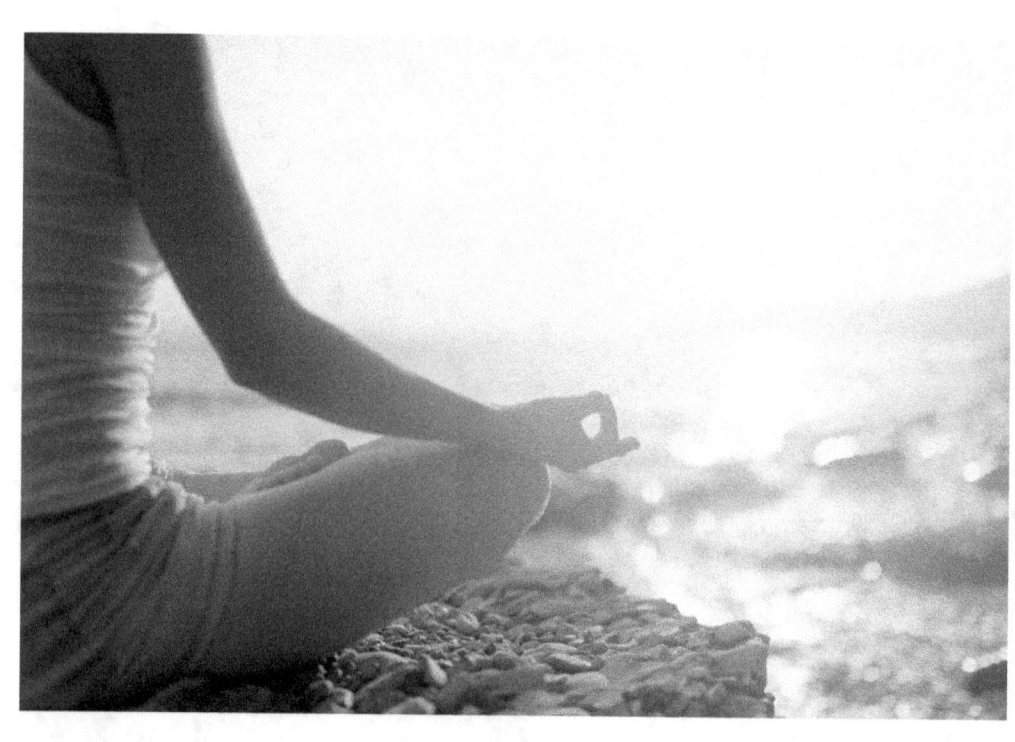

Class 5
Durga Devi

- Opening Prayers
- Neck rolls, five times in each direction, right then left.
- Stretch the ear to shoulder with corresponding hand creating resistance.
- Half Moon, ardha chandrasana
- Three slow Sun salutations, surya namaskar, runner's pose, into extended side triangle, utthita parsva konasana, into chair, utkasana.
- Wide standing forward bend with an arched back, prasarita padottanasana
- Hero, virasana, swaying and lifting from left to center and right to center.
- Seated fan knees toward chest and then the floor. Then place heal on thighs and fold over leg, then come up and twist forward, opposite hand to foot.
- Camel, ustrasana variation with one hand on foot looking over that shoulder
- Cat/Cow variation, ardha dhanurasana, cross ankle over back of other leg and with the opposite hand grab foot and lift.
- Planks, caturanga dandasana into downward dogs, adho mukta svanasana with fluid mobility into child's pose, balasana
- Classic half locust, ardha shalabhasana, shalabhasana, full locust hands on ground, one leg and then both legs.
- Classic boat, navasana, thumbs tough arms and head in alignment.
- Leg raises with foot flexion slowly, working with a count of 10-12.
- Bridge, setu bandhasana, with shoulder adjustments
- Rod pose, dandasana, carry leg as if a baby, then place heal next to pelvis, fold forward, both sides
- Seated boat, navasana, start with legs tucked into the body. Lift one leg and then the other and then both legs together.
- Tip toe balance pose, flower, pushpasana, with hand at the heart.
- Savasana
- Meditation:
- Rhythmic breathing, Savitri pranayama. Inhale, hold, exhale, and hold to all the same count.
- 4-1-4-1
- 4-2-4-2
- 4-3-4-3
- 4-4-4-4
- Shambhavi mudra, Thumbs on ear flaps, first finger just below eyebrows, second finger lightly touch nostrils, third finger at skin flap above mouth, forth finger rests on chin. An experience of NOD, the cosmic sound of the universe.
- Closing prayers

Class 6
Sat Yam

- Opening prayers
- Cat/ Cow stretch, vidalasana
- Interlace hands behind the head, alternate opposite elbow to opposite knee. Straighten legs and cross to opposite side of body, on floor, turn head towards foot on floor. Repeat sequence several times and then repeat sequence on the other sides of the body.
- Pigeon stretches, eka pada rajakapotasana
- Downward dog on toes, adho mukta svavasana
- Forward bend, uttanasana
- Reverse swan dive
- Half moon stretches, ardha chandrasana
- Reverse swan dive into extended side flank, utthita parsva konasana
- Runner's stretches, toes engaged
- Downward dog, adho mukta svansana
- Forward bend, uttanasana into chair, utkatasana
- Warrior I, virabhadrasana I
- Cobra, bhujangasana three times
- Locust half and full locust, ardha shalabhasana, shalabhasana
- Bow, dhanurasana, two times hold, feet then ankles
- Boat, navasana, two times
- One arm balancing pose, vasistasana, lying on left side double up mat end and place forearm there with other hand on the floor, lift over shoulder up with the hips, place arm at side. Both sides two times.
- Lift arm over leg and clasp other hand, rock the hip out to the side.
- Revolved bound head to knee, parivrtta janu sirsasana. Start with putting a little pressure on hip/leg, and then add in one arm at a time, looking over shoulder.
- Gentle partner rocking in supported shoulder stand, salamba sarvangasana. Nice and easy lift up three times, then lift legs up to ceiling and lift head and neck and drop into boat, navasana.
- Lotus on back, supta padmasana, both sides two times
- Savasana
- Yoga Nidra; Going into the center of the heart, the heart of hearts, seat of all transformation. Affirmations in inverted Namaste' Mudra, Temple breathing. Anchor awareness on unconditional love, bliss, compassion.
- Meditation:
- Blue/White light

- 16-18 inches above head. Pure Love.
- Left hand is lifted palm up at heart center; right hand rests on knee fingers touch the ground, Mother Earth.
- Working with seed sounds, SAT, truth, YAM, heart, eight times and then silence.
- Closing Prayers

Class 7
Sitting in Truth

- Cat/ Cow, vidalasana
- Downward dog, adho mukha svanasana
- Pigeon with arms clasped behind back, eka pada rajakapotanasana
- Downward dog, adho mukha svanasana
- Half moon, ardha chandrasana
- Slow sun salutations, surya namaskar, lowering body into plank, caturanga dandasana rather than cobra, bhujangasana and several planks, caturanga dandasana.
- Partner tree, vrikasana
- Lord Krishna's pose - natavarasana
- Half locust, ardha shalabhasana, two times
- Full locust, shalabhasana, two times
- Cobra with arms clasped behind back, bhujangasana two times
- Half bow, opposite arm to foot with other arm on floor, ardha dhanurasana, two times
- One arm balancing pose, vasisthanasa, two times both sides
- Full bow, dhanurasana, wide knees
- Frog stretch looking over one shoulder at a time, mandukasana
- Knee drops, two times
- Leg lifts, single and then both times while lying on the back
- Wing releasing poses lifting neck to see navel, pavanamuktasana
- Savasana
- Yoga Nidra
- Meditation:
- Blue/White light, following the sound of the breath with the SAT YAM mantra
- Closing Prayers

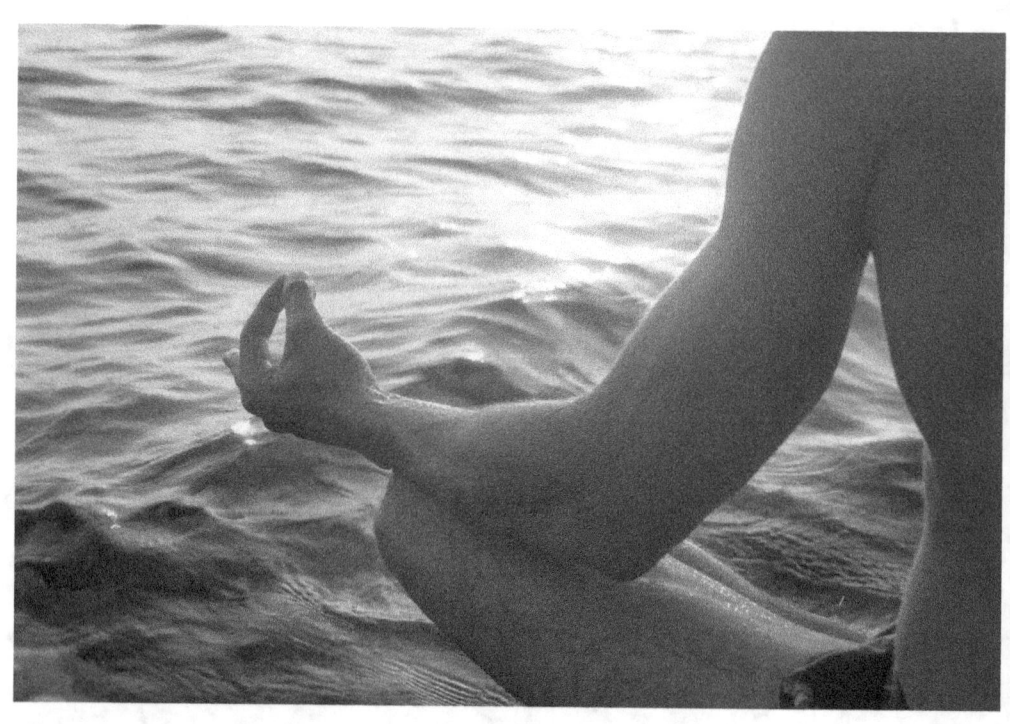

Class 8
So Ham

- Opening prayers
- Seated neck rolls, drawing chin in to sturnal notch over to shoulder and then look up with eyes.
- Downward dog with bent knees, adho mukta svanasana
- Pigeon stretches, eka pada rajakapotasana, regular and then open knee to side of mat, foot in center.
- Half-moon, ardha chandrasana, two times each side
- Slow sun salutations, surya namaskar
- Water wheel, three times
- Cobra, bhujangasana, two times
- Half locust, ardha shalabhasana two times
- Full locust, shalabhasana two times
- Child's pose, balasana, wide knees
- Rabbit, sasagasana
- Head to knee with fingers clasped, janu sirsasana
- One arm one leg balance, vasisthanasa, two times each side
- Leg lifts, bring knees to chest and then place one leg on ground, raise leg off ground eight inches from floor, slowly lower other leg to floor.
- Savasana
- Yoga Nidra
- Meditation:
- Lift mulabhanda 8 times and focus breath on SO HAM mantra
- From Satchidananda Ashram-Yogaville:
- Asato Maa Sad Gamaya
- Tamaso Maa Jyotir Gamaya
- Mrityor Maa Amritam Gamaya.
- Lead us from the unreal to the Real
- Lead us from darkness to Light
- Lead us from fear of death
- To knowledge of Immortality.
- Closing Prayers

Class 9
Goddesses

- Opening prayers
- Lobular Breathing - Seated pranayama, gyana mudra with thumbs in, thumbs up and thumbs out.
- Check to see which lobes open.
- Nadi shodhana
- Chandra bhedana
- Seated in hero, virasana, neck rolls from sturnal notch to left, clockwise two and to the right, counterclockwise, two times.
- Ear drops to shoulder, two times
- Cat/ Cow, vidalasana eight times
- Half-moon, ardha chandrasana, two times
- Windmill breathing, three times
- Forward bend, uttanasana
- Triangle variation, trikonasana, arm at hip, stretch other arm up, bend, drop neck, release arm. Neck together, two times each side
- Intense warrior
- Runner's pose into lank, caturanga dandasana into downward dog, adho mukta svanasana (bent knees), inchworm, ashtangasana. Repeat and add a child's pose, balasana, three times.
- Diamond Pose
- Frog stretch, one leg at a time.
- Half locust stretch, ardha shalabhasana
- Half locust variation, ardha shalabhasana
- Full locust, shalabhasana
- Half bow, ardha dhanurasana, using same arm, same leg
- Child's pose, balasana into diamond pose
- Crane pose, bakasana with knees balancing on the arms
- Savasana
- Yoga Nidra
- Song....
- "Saraswati, Maha Laxashmi, Durga Devi, Namaha"
- Meditation
- Meditate on one aspect of the song, one quality of the Goddess.
- Closing prayers

Class 10
Children of the Light

- Opening prayers
- Cat/Cow, vidalasana
- Cat/Cow, vidalasana, with all three bandhas; jalandhara, uddiyana, mula bandha.
- Plank, caturanga dandasana
- Downward dog, adho mukha svanasana
- Pigeon, eka pada rajakapotasana
- Sun salutations, surya namaskar, with extended side flank, utthita parsva konasana, Warrior II, virabhadrasana II, and half moon, ardha candrasana
- Dancer both arm variations, Lord Natarajasana pose
- Opposite legs up the wall variation, viparita karani
- Tranquility pose
- Fish, matsyasana
- Bull poses with a forward bend
- Lincoln logs, legs stacked with a forward bend
- Mermaid leg stretches
- Revolved stomach poses, jathara parivartanasana
- Savasana
- Yoga Nidra, again focusing on the heart
- Song...
- "I am a child of the Light,
- I serve the Light,
- The Light and I are one being,
- I am protected, supported, and illumined by the Light,
- The Light and I are one being."
- Meditation:
- Namaste' Mudra Series by Sandra Kozak

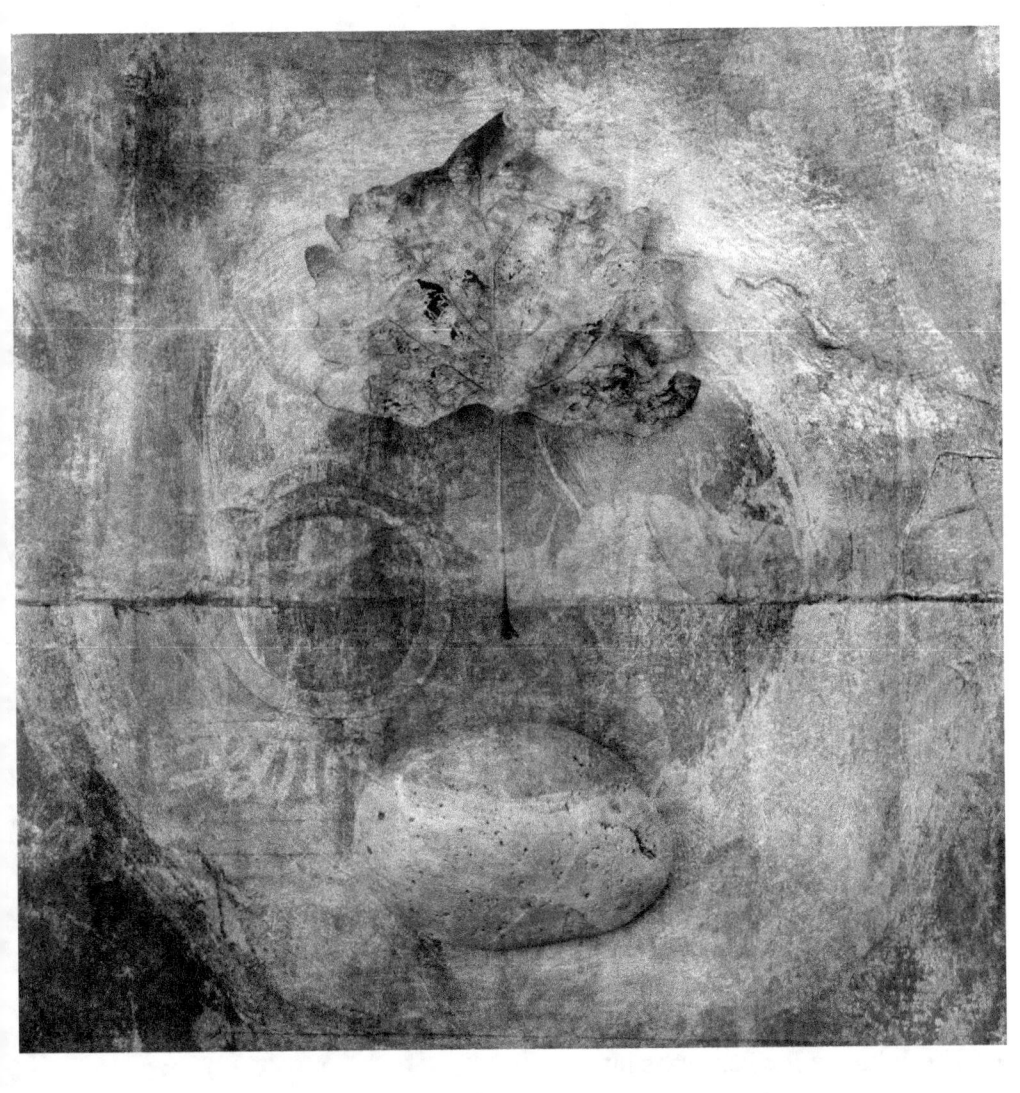

Class 11
The River

- Opening prayers
- Kapalabhati pranayama exercise
- Cat/Cow warm up, vidalasana
- Cat/Cow holding all the three most important bandhas; jalandara, uddiyana, mula bandha
- Plank, caturanga dandasana
- Downward dog, adho mukha svanasana
- Pigeon, eka pada rajakapotasana
- Pigeon, eka pada rajakapotasana, with body resting on bent knee, opposite arm rotates behind, looking over shoulder
- Half-moon, ardha chandrasana
- Runner's stretch
- Forward fold over front leg, both legs extended, parsvottanasana
- Repeat, again with partners and blocks.
- Splits, hanumanasana
- Cobra/locust variations, from cobra hands touch at the small of back and lift. Neck turns one way from the small of back. Hands and arms rotate and lift forward above, head level. Repeat sequence on both sides.
- Then arms/hands rotate in a diamond in front above head and then the arms open, as in superman.
- Seated spinal twists, holding one hand on knee, the other on foot.
- Savasana
- Silent meditation
- Ram Dass Song:
- "The river is flowing
- Flowing and growing
- The river is flowing
- Back to the sea.
- Mother Earth carry me
- The child I will will always be
- Mother carry me
- Back to the sea."
- Closing prayers

Class 12
Om Mani Padme Hume

- Opening prayers
- Energy block releasing sequence
- Cat/Cow, vidalasana
- Cat/Cow with bandhas
- Cat/Cow with arms/legs extended, vidalasana
- Downward dog, adho mukha svanasana
- Plank, caturanga dandasana
- Downward dog, adho mukha svanasana
- Plank, caturanga dandasana
- Pigeon, eka pada rajakapotasana variation with one knee bent one leg behind. Look at fingertips of one arm as it rotates to leg stretched behind.
- Reversed warrior into warrior II, virabhadrasana II, two times each side.
- Block exercises between legs engaging mula bandha/apana vayu
- Tree pose, vrksasana, at calf, at thigh, two times
- Hero, virasana
- Half locust, ardha shalabhasana, variation, bend one knee at a time, sole of foot towards ceiling, raise thigh up.
- Full locust, shalabhasana, two times each side
- Classical cobra, bhujangasana, two times
- Child's pose, balasana
- Bridge, setu bandhasana, with block, two angles of block; skinny and thick sides
- Bridge, setu bandhasana, on block with legs extended towards ceiling, one at time and then both.
- Revolving stomach pose, jathara parivartanasana, with knees bent
- Wind relieving pose, pavanamuktasana
- Savasana
- Yoga Nidra, beginning with right toe and ending with the heart.
- Meditation:
- OM MANI PADME HUME
- Outloud and silent
- Closing prayers

Class 13
Longevity

- Opening prayers
- Full yogic breath – attention placed at belly
- Cat/Cow, vidalasana seated kapalabhati with breath retention focused at ajna chakra
- Seated twists, hands on shoulders, inhale left, exhale right
- Shoulder drops with breath retention
- Seated twists, inhale left, exhale right, hand to opposite foot looking over shoulder, again breath retention focused on ajna chakra
- Prasarita padottanasana variations, legs together and out to the side in splits
- Rod pose, dandasana, with chest lifted, releases tension in upper back
- Half boat, ardha navasana with partner
- Anantasana, Vishnu's couch variations and warmups plus partner assist
- Splits, Pose dedicated to Hanuman, Hanumanasana
- Runner's stretch
- Forward bend, uttanasana
- Bridge, setu bandhasana
- Wind relieving leg stretches with toes pointed and opposite leg extended, pavanamuktasana.
- Knee drops
- Savasana
- Yoga Nidra; drawing on the qualities of the heart, love, compassion, and strength.
- Song/Meditation:
- "Om Dhum Durgai Namaha
- "Om Krim Kali Kai Namaha"
- Closing prayers

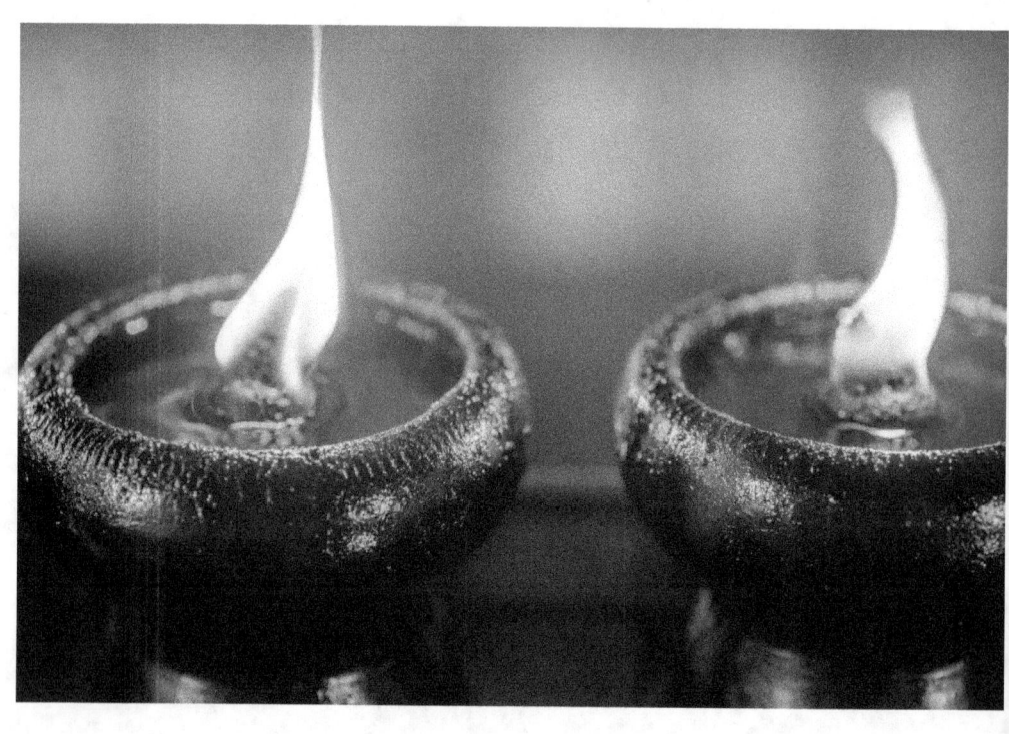

Class 14
My Heart's Song

- Opening prayers
- Cat/Cow, vidalasana
- Downward dog, adho mukha svanasana
- Plank, caturanga dandasana
- Pigeon, eka pada rajakapotasana, variation with arms stretched and interlaced behind body, three rounds
- Downward dog, adho mukha svanasana
- Plank, caturanga dandasana
- Camel, ustrasana, stretches into half-moon, ardha chandrasana seated stretches
- Runner's balancing stretches
- Downward dog, adho mukta svanasana, at wall
- Extended side flank, parsva konasana, at wall, two times each side
- Extended triangle, utthita trikonasana, with block at wall, two times each side
- Inverted Pose, viparita karani at wall with pressure on the bottom of the feet from partner
- Shoulderstand, sarvangasana, stretches at wall
- Reclining bound angle, supta baddha konasana
- Cobra, bhujangasana, with hands on buttocks
- Half locust leg stretches, ardha shalabhasana
- Half bow, ardha dhanurasana, with same and opposite hand to foot
- Bow, dhanurasana
- High cobra, bhujangasana, two times
- Child's pose, balasana, wide knee variation
- Seated twists, marichyasana
- Savasana
- Yoga Nidra
- Song...
- "Listen; listen to my heart's song,
- Listen; listen to my heart's song,
- I will never forsake you,
- I will never forget you." 4 times
- Closing prayers

Class 15
Vashista Pranayamas

- Opening prayers
- Hip openers on back
- Vashista pranayamas as taught by Dr. Vasant Lad, Cockabrushundi taught Vashista these pranayamas
1. Anuloma Viloma, 20 times, 2–3-minute rest of Kevala Kumbaka
2. Kapalabhati, quick diaphragm breathing, 60, 2–3-minute rest
3. Bhramari, 12, 2–3-minute rest. Shoulder circles both directions, raise arms and sway from side to side
4. Ujjayi, 12, opens crown charka
- Savasana – complete relaxation with focus on abdominal breath and downward gaze, eyes sink back to the sockets, relaxed tongue, surrender to floor.
- Closing prayers

MAHAMRITYUNJAYA MANTRA:
SACRED MANTRA FOR HEALING
AND PROTECTION as chanted at Satchidananda Ashram-Yogaville

OM Tryambakam Yajaamahe One,
Sugandhim Pushti Vardhanam
Urvaarukamiva Bandhanaan
be cut Mrityor Muksheeya Maamritaat
(3 Times)

We worship the All-Seeing

Fragrant, nourishes bounteously
From fear of death may we free,
To realize Immortality.

Class 16
Marmani Work

- Opening prayers
- Vasishta pranayamas
- Standing warmups
- From mountain pose, tadasana, lengthen neck upwards and then look down tucking chin in, then look over right side, chest forward, neck/head towards shoulders. Then look over to the left side.
- Inhale arms overhead, twist and squat to right and inhale again to center.
- Inhale arms overhead and twist and squat to left.
- As you inhale upwards press heals of hands outwards.
- Half-moon, ardha chandrasana, adding one arm and then two, exhale pressing heals of hands aware from you.
- Windmill breathing standing, arms rotate forwards and backwards.
- Extended forward bend with legs apart, prasarita padottanasana
- Twisting from this forward bend with arm/elbow on ground, both sides
- Extended forward bend, utthita parsvottanasana, legs one leg distance apart, head resting on the ground.
- Revolved triangle, parivrtta trikonasana, with block, two times both sides
- Revolved side plank, parivrtta parsvakonasana, two times with knee on ground and then lifted.
- Flower poses, pushpasana, with wide knees
- Crane pose, bakasana
- Partner Marma Cikitsa, healing through the energy points
- Closing prayers

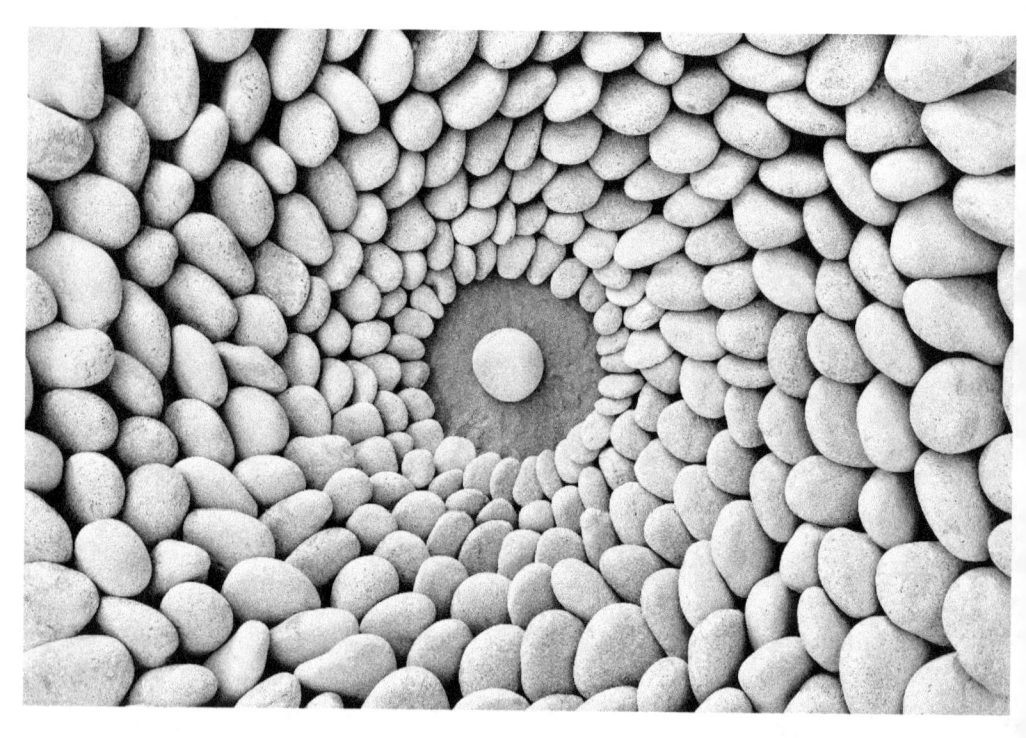

Class 17
AUM & Gayatri Mantra

- Opening prayers
- Lecture on **AUM & Gayatri Mantra**
- From a triangle it all began. The triangle broke open and the sound **AUM** was created.

The symbol and its wisdom:
1. waking consciousness
2. dreaming consciousness
3. sleeping consciousness
4. transpersonal consciousness
5. cosmic consciousness
   - 1, 2, 3 = gunas/gods
   - Brahma, Vishnu, Shiva
   - Sattva, Tamas, Rajas
   - **GAYATRI MANTRA: Rig-Veda (3.62.10)**
   - Om bhur bhuvah svah
   - tat savitur varenyam
   - bhargo devasya dhimahi
   - dhiyo yo nah prachodayat
   - Let us contemplate the wonderous Spirit of the divine creator of the earthly, atmospheric, and celestial spheres, may He/She direct our minds towards attainment of Dharma, Artha, Kama and Moksha. (Virtues, wealth, desires, and liberation)
   - Asana portion:
   - 5 Tibetans
   - Bridge, setu bandhasana, with knees together, shoulders descended, two times
   - Wind releasing, pavanamuktasana
   - Revolved stomach pose, jathara parivartanasana, two times, lower legs slower to floor
   - Wind releasing, pavanamuktasana
   - Savasana
   - Yoga Nidra
   - Seated prayers/Meditation:
   - "Dear God, you are inside of me
   - Within my very breath
   - Within each bird, each mighty mountain
   - Your sweet touch reaches everything
   - and I am well protected.
   - Thank you, God,
   - for this beautiful day before me.

- May joy, love, peace, and compassion
- Be apart of my life
- and all those around me on this day.

I am healing and I am healed."
By Dr. Vasant Lad
Closing prayers

Class 18
Flexibility

- Opening prayers
- Shoulder work
- One shoulder rotating forward, then shoulder rotates backwards. Repeat exercise several times and then switch shoulder rolling directions.
- Shoulder lifts
- Shoulder twists
- Extending through arms, inhaling up, and then releasing shoulders back down on an inhale.
- Partner assists, fold forward with arms interlaced allow partner to give a slight lift and pull.
- At wall, place hands with middle finger pointing up, rotate humorous bone up
- At wall, arm rotations and twists
- Extended side flank, utthita parsva konasana
- Triangle, trikonasana
- Extended side flank series, utthita parsva konasana, eight times
- Triangle, trikonasana
- Classic cobra, bhujangasana
- Cobra with fingers interlaced on back, bhujangasana
- Locust variation, shalabhasana, knees bent, feet touch, arms lift up on back
- Wind relieving pose, pavanamuktasana
- On back, raise legs and arms into the air, lower arms to the floor, release legs to the sides, five times
- Wind relieving pose, pavanamuktasana
- Half knee down twist, supta matysendrasana, both sides
- Savasana
- Yoga Nidra, toes to heart
- Meditation
- Bhastrika, Bellow's breathe, two times up to 2 minutes only
- Closing prayers

Class 19
Meditation for Abundance

- Opening prayers
- Pranayama seated in thunderbolt, virasana
- Cat/Cow, vidalasana
- Twists inhale left, exhale right
- Shoulder drops
- Child's pose, balasana
- Downward dog, adho mukha svanasana
- Forward bend, uttanasana
- Half-moon, ardha chandrasana
- Backbend/forward bend, uttanasana
- Shoulder stretches at wall with blocks in thighs
- Standing boat, navasana at wall, back arched, four times
- Shoulderstand, sarvangasana, variations, slowly, four times
- Inverted pose, viparita karani
- One arm, one leg balance, Vasisthasana, both sides
- Frog stretch, mandukasana, one leg at a time, both legs together
- Lying on back, takes hands in Tadaka/Tagari Mudra on belly inhale, exhale, retention, massage stomach
- Lying on back, twist one knee over the other, both sides
- Savasana
- Yoga Nidra
- Meditation for Abundance:
- "Om Shrim, Om Hrim, Om Shrim,
- Kamala, Kamalayla,
- Proceda, Proceda, Shrim, Hrim, Shrim,
- Om Shri Maha Laxshmi
- Deveye Namaha."
- Closing prayers

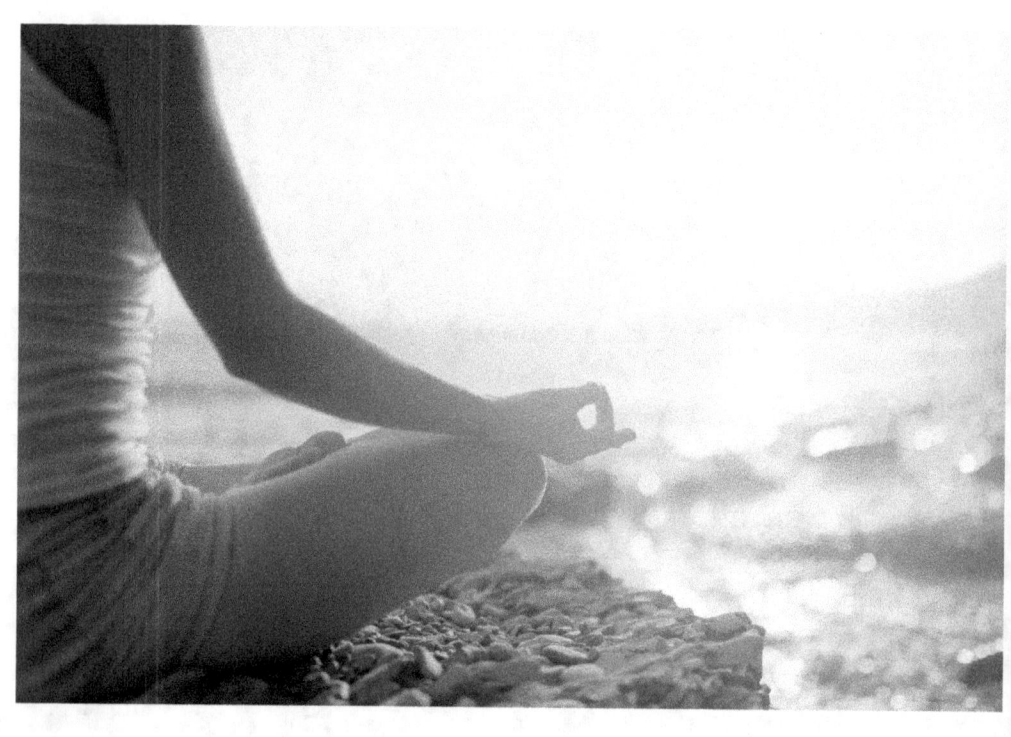

Class 20
Yoga for the Eyes

- Opening prayers
- Eye exercises, nethra vayayayam
- Cat/Cow, vidalasana
- Puppy dog stretch
- Child's pose, balasana
- Downward dog on toes, adho mukha svanasana
- Child's pose, balasana
- Downward dog, adho mukha svanasana
- Pigeon, left then right, eka pada rajakapotasana
- Downward dog, walk hands into uttanasana
- Half-moon, ardha chandrasana, into breathing sequence
- Chair poses series, utkatasana
- Chair, utkatanasana into suspension bridge into one leg raises into warrior I, virabhadrasana I into triangle, trikonasana into extended side flank, utthita parsva konasana into forward bend, uttanasana.
- Second time adding in warrior II, virabhadrasana II.
- Rest on back, savasana
- Bridge, setu bandhasana, two times
- Add in block first time, leg lifts one at a time and then both legs.
- Twists on back, supta matysendrasana
- Tadagi Mudra, inhale exhale massage stomach
- Savasana
- Yoga Nidra
- Pranayama
- Bhramari, inhale female bee sound, exhale male bee sound
- Closing prayers

Class 21
Deep Relaxation

- Opening prayers
- Cat/Cow, vidalasana
- Puppy dog stretch
- Cat/Cow arm/leg extensions, vidalasana
- Child's pose, balasana
- Plank, caturanga dandasana
- Downward dog, adho mukha svanasana
- Planks, caturanga dandasana, into child's pose, balasana, two times
- Hero's pose, virasana, into leg foot stretches drawing one leg forward, lift leg and draw straight leg into lunge, three times each side
- Intense Leg Stretch, utthita parsvottanasana, with block
- Warrior II, virabhadrasana II, lunge with block, on outside of ankle
- Triangle, trikonasana, with block
- Boat, navasana, with fingers interlaced, three times
- Frog stretches, each side, mandukasana
- Locust, shalabhasana, variation with knees bent, feet touch in a triangle
- Wind relieving pose, pavanamuktasana
- With knees bent to chest, rock in slow circles to both sides
- Lift chest/head to right then to center, then left to chest
- Ankles over each other for twist
- Savasana
- Yoga Nidra
- Vashista pranayamas
- Anuloma Viloma 20
- Kapalabhati 60
- Bhramari 12
- Ujjayi 12
- Meditation
- Closing prayers

Class 22
OM MA

- Opening prayers
- Standing warm-ups
- Shoulder work
- Neck rolls
- Squat into twist into pulse, two times each side
- Half-moon, ardha chandrasana, with thumbs interlaced, two times each side
- Bow and arrow breathing
- Heart chakra breathing
- T.V.K. Desikachar sequence.... Warrior breathing with legs, arms and torso in Windmill breathing with breath retention
- Forward bend, uttanasana, with block
- Partner assist, hands to back of hamstrings
- Half locust, ardha shalabhasana, two times
- Boat variations, navasana, three times
- Vishnu's couch, anantasana
- Downward dog, adho mukha svanasana, into child's poses, balasana, sequence
- One point Hara exercise, tummy in, tailbone under, fill the Hara with breath, 360*
- Partner shoulder stand, salamba sarvangasana, in rocking motion
- Opposite arm/leg raises
- Savasana
- Yoga Nidra
- Meditation:
- OM MA
- Closing prayers

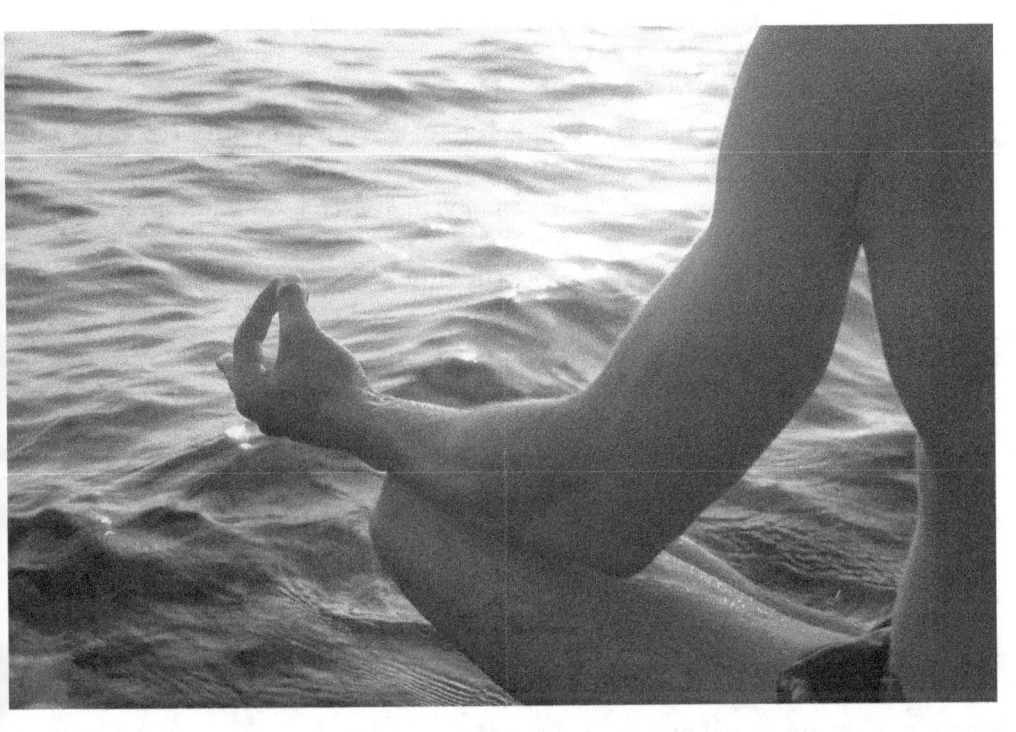

Class 23
Love in All Things

- Opening prayers
- Pelvis/hip opener class
- Lying on back, one knee at a time into chest, then extend leg onto floor, both sides
- Take a tie to the ball of the foot extend through bones, flat foot at ceiling, both feet
- Then rotate hip/leg towards shoulders with tie.
- West stretch, pashchimottanasana, full forward bend with tie, allows hips to lift off floor.
- Eight times half boat, ardha navasana, arm at 45*. Lift head and keep arm angled.
- Classic full locust, shalabhasana, three times
- Frog stretches, two times each side
- Child's pose, balasana, with toes being stretched
- Downward dog, adho mukha svanasana, on toes, slowly release heals
- Child's pose, balasana, three times
- Rabbit pose, sasagasana
- Partner assisted shoulder stand, salamba sarvangasana
- Cat/ cow, vidalasana, variation, cross ankle over other and lift opposite hand/foot
- Revolved stomach pose, jathara parivartanasana, two times with tie
- Savasana
- Yoga Nidra
- Shamanic journey: Love in All Things
- Song...
- "I am a child of the Light,
- I serve the Light,
- The Light and I are one being,
- I am a child of the Light,
- I am protected, supported, and illumined by the Light,
- The Light and I are one being."
- Closing prayers

Class 24
Yoga Nidra of the Heart

- Opening prayers
- Standing warm-ups, uddiyana bandha, agni sardoti
- Windmeal breathing exercises, forward and backward, two times
- Half-moon, ardha chandrasana two times
- Slow sun salutations, surya namaskar, with extended side angle, utthita parsva konasana, no inch worm, ashtangasana, pull back into child's pose, balasana, and then hold chair, utkatasana after sequence, three times
- Warrior II, virabhadrasana II
- Lunge into hold hand to foot, then stretch opposite hand into triangle, trikonasana, two times
- Half locust, ardha shalabhasana, two times
- Half boat, ardha navasana, opposite hand foot, two times
- Full boat, navasana, two times
- Cobra, bhujangasana, two times without use of hands
- Rabbit pose, sasagasana, tuck chin for greater stretch
- Wind relieving pose, pavanamuktasana, on back open knees to floor, two times
- Stretch one leg towards floor while on back and then the other, two times
- Navasana, release of legs while on back, twist, readjust ear, hips move up.
- Savasana
- Yoga Nidra of the Heart
- Vasishta Pranayamas
- Anuloma Viloma 20
- Kapalabhati 60
- Bhramari 12
- Ujjayi 12
- Closing prayers

Class 25
Golden/White Light

- Opening prayers
- Vata balancing warm-ups
- Half moon, ardha candrasana on knees
- Runner stretches into planks, caturanga dandasana into downward dog, adho mukha svanasana into high cobras, bhujangasana into child's pose, balasana into extended forward intense leg; utthita parsvottanasana stretches into pigeon stretches.
- Cow's head pose, gomukasana
- Half locust, ardha shalabhasana, variation with opposite leg supporting knee
- Still crocodile, makarasana
- High cobras, bhujangasana looking over shoulders, tiryaka bhujangasana
- While seated, arms up in a triangle, stretch elbows towards floor
- Bound angle, baddha konasana
- Rock the baby
- Stringing the bow, dhanurakarshanasana
- Lotus, padmasana
- Hidden lotus, baddha padmasana
- Lotus with blocks under hands, lolasana
- Seated navasana variations, legs together, legs apart
- Viparita karani or shoulderstand, sarvangasana
- Fish, matsyasana
- Wind relieving pose, pavanamuktasana
- Savasana
- Yoga Nidra
- Meditation:
- Golden/White light pyramid including those names of people we love.
- Ram Dass Song:
- "The river is flowing
- Flowing and growing
- The river is flowing
- Back to the sea.
- Mother Earth carry me
- The child I will always be
- Mother carry me
- Back to the sea."
- Closing prayers

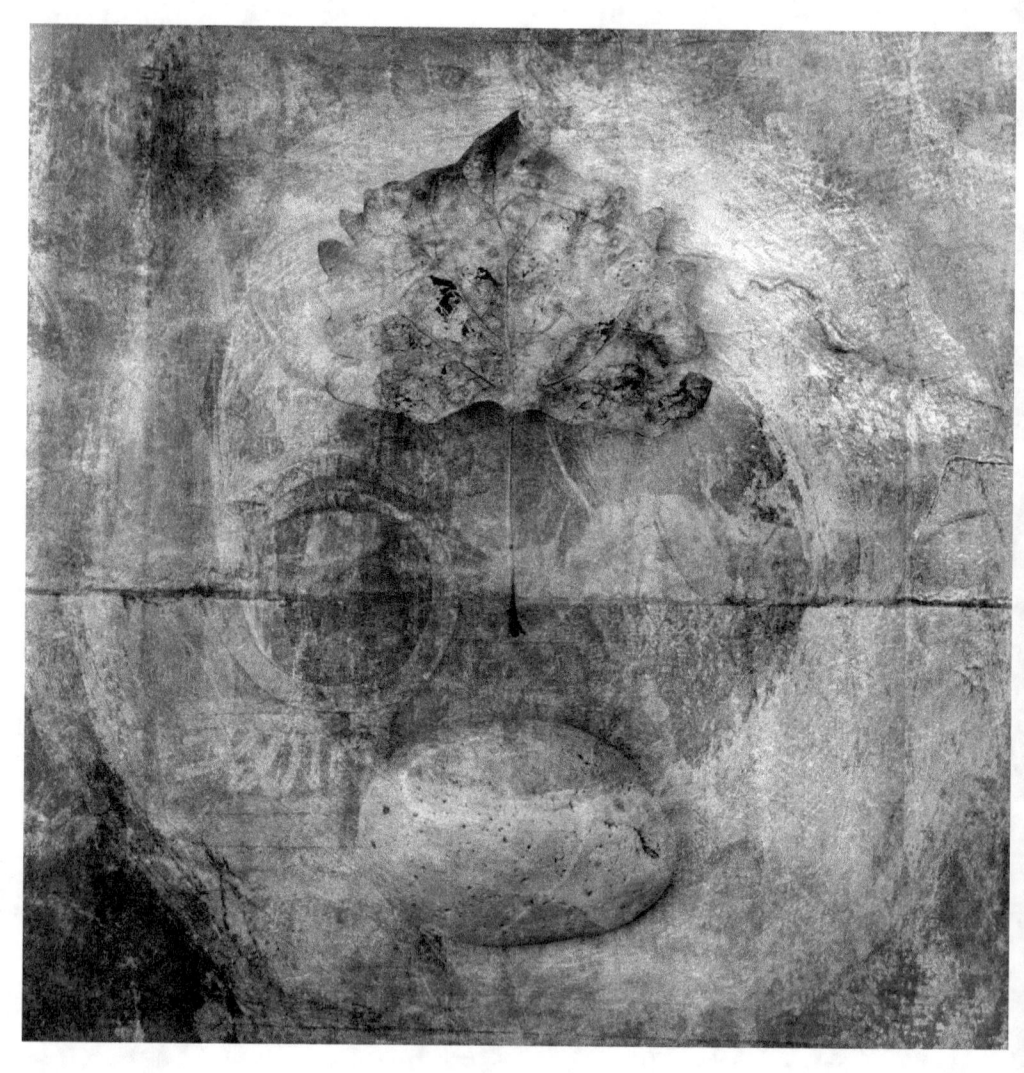

Class 26
Bija Mantras

- Opening prayers
- Restorative class
- Legs up the wall or lying on back, utthita eka padmasana, eyes closed
- Breathe up back body, exhale down front body
- Breathe up front body, exhale down back body
- Bridge, setu bandhasana, vinyasana sequence at wall or with bent knees on back
- Breathe into seat of kapha
- On hand and knees, lengthen one leg at a time behind you, repetition of four
- Leg stretches, intense forward one leg stretches, utthita parsvottanasana
- Windmill breathing
- Standing in mountain, tadasana, raise arms up and twist in one direction, bend in towards toes. On the other side repeat the sequence.
- Shoulder stretches, hands join together at heart, resist stretch
- Downward dog, adho mukha svanasana into plank, caturanga dandasana into child's pose, balasana, several times rolling through
- Forward bend, uttanasana
- Neck rolls, atlas/axis rotations in each direction
- Mt. Kalish, slowly around the mountain
- Pigeon, eka pada rajakapotasana, sequence down on floor, arms extended, look all the way up and all the way down.
- Forward bend, prasarita padottasana, with legs open wide, arms twisted behind back
- Squat with eagle arms head bends forward.
- Half locust, ardha shalabhasana, arms under body, two times
- Full locust, shalabhasana, two times
- Classical cobra, bhujangasana, two times
- Frog stretch, each side
- Full bow, dhunrasana, two times
- Child's pose, balasana, into hare, sasagasana
- Leg lifts, drawing one knee in, set of four, lowering leg two inches off floor, both sides of body
- Lying on back do belly breathing again
- Anitasana, Vishnu's couch, two times each side
- Abdominal massage on back, hands moving into pelvis
- Leg lifts, with legs together, lift head/neck off floor
- Reclining bound angle, supta baddha konasana
- Wind relieving pose, pavanamuktasana
- Half knee down twist, supta matysendrasana, both sides

- Savasana
- Yoga Nidra
- Bija mantra meditation
- Seed sound, color, chakra, experience
- LAM, Muladhara, Earth, RED
- VAM, Svadhistana, Water, ORANGE
- RAM, Manipurna, Fire, YELLOW
- YAM, Anahata, Air, GREEN
- HAM, Vishuddha, Ether, BLUE
- SAM/KSHAM, Ajna, Consciousness, INDIGO
- AUM, Sahasrara, Bliss, VIOLET
- Closing prayers

Class 27
Silence

- Opening prayers
- Seated warm-ups
- Imagine holding on to a beach ball while seated. Arch back and release forward.
- Seated draw one arm forward, twist torso and follow arm around with arm, both sides
- Staff poses, dandasana, shake legs out
- Draw one leg over thigh, interlace fingers through toes, and spread toes.
- Rotate ankles in both directions
- Revolved head over knee, parivrtta janu sirsasana
- Gate pose, parighasana
- Rock the baby
- Half bow, ardha dhuranasana variations, lift chest as opposite arm stretches forward, other arm/leg join, both sides.
- Half locust stretch, ardha shalabhasana
- Full classical locust, shalabhasana
- Classical cobra, bhujangasana, two times, lift arms from floor
- Cobra, bhujangasana, hand next to chest, two times
- Full bow, dhanurasana
- Child's pose, balasana
- Downward dog, adho mukha svanasana, several minutes
- Plank, caturanga dandasana
- Pigeon pose, eka pada rajakapotasana, arms flat on floor and then under shoulders
- Mermaid pose
- Rock pose
- Hands under arms in rock pose
- Lift legs and bring towards face in rock pose
- Wind relieving pose, pavanamuktasana
- Legs at a 90* angle from body, partner pushes on feet, urdhava prasaritta padasana
- Wind relieving pose, pavanamuktasana
- Twists
- Boat, navasana on back
- Savasana
- Yoga Nidra from the Bihar School of Yoga
- Four purifications:
- Nodi Shodana, Kapalbhati, Agni Sardoti, Ashwini mudra
- Silent meditation
- Closing prayer

Class 28
Life Dancer

- Opening prayers
- Energy block releasing sequence
- Breath of Arjuna
- Affirmations in inverted Namaste' Mudra, Temple breathing
- "I am," "I am one," "I am one with the Universe" At root, at heart, at crown.
- Two very slow sun salutations, surya namaskar
- Second with pigeon, eka pada rajakapotasana, woven in
- Two very fast sun salutations, surya namaskar with high cobra, bhujangasana
- Rest on back
- Half locust stretches with knees bent, two times
- Half locust, ardha salabhasana, two times
- Full locust, salabhasana, two times
- Half boat, ardha navasana, two times
- Full boat, navasana, two times
- Half bow, ardha dhanurasana, cross one leg at ankle, opposite hand holds foot and lift leg upwards, two times each side
- Child's pose, balasana, wrap arms around shoulders
- Draw knees into chest with stomach muscles
- Legs at 90*angle from body, rotate through ankles/feet, urdhva prasarita padasana
- Half knee down twist, supta matysendrasana
- Wind relieving pose, pavanamuktasana
- Savasana
- Yoga Nidra, focusing on the heart
- Meditation, at brow point, ajna chakra
- Hands in Deer, Tatva mudra – thumb, middle, and ring fingers touch lightly. Index and pinky finger extend out, on both hands.
- Savitri Pranayama
- 4-1-4-1
- 4-2-4-2
- 4-3-4-3
- 4-4-4-4
- Closing prayers

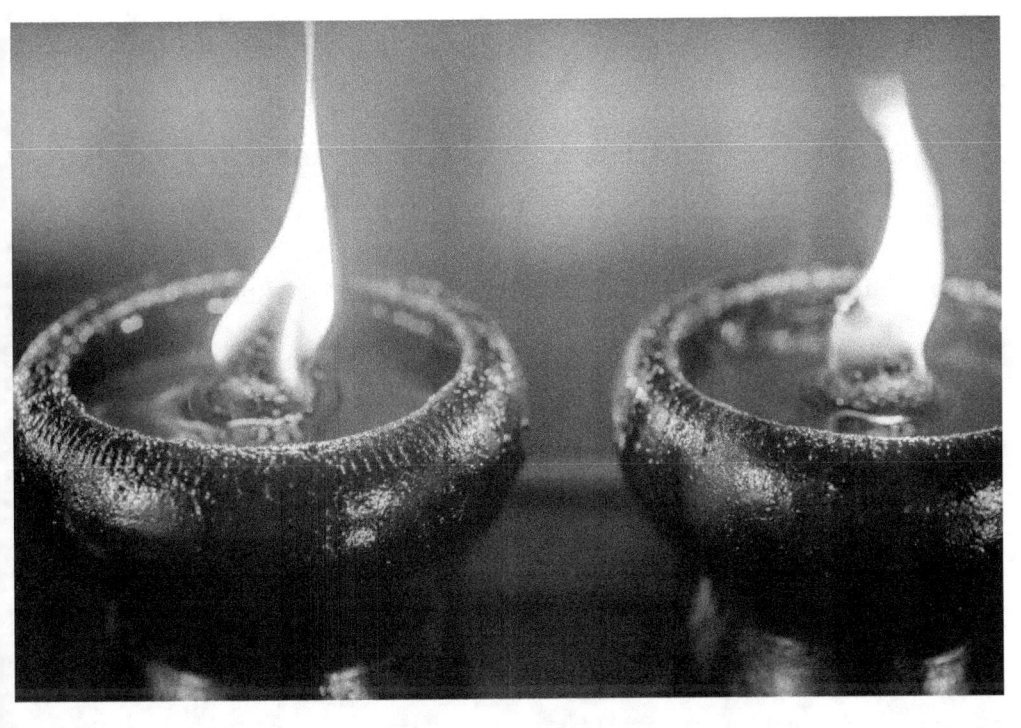

BIBLIOGRAPHY

"Excerpted with permission from *The Daily* by Dr. Vasant Lad, originally published in *Ayurveda Today,* Volume 6, Number 3. Copyright © 1993. All Rights Reserved."

Dass, Baba Hari. *Ashtanga Yoga Primer.* Santa Cruz: Sri Rama Publishing, 1981.

Guru, Ram Dass. Song.

Hansen, Patricia. Lectures and Yoga handouts. Denver, 2004-2005.

Knox. Hansa. *Comtemplative Hatha Teacher Training Manual.* Denver: Self Published, 2001.

Kozak, Summerfield Sandra. *Namaste Mudra Series.* Phoenix: International Yoga Studies, 2001.

Lad, Vasant. *AyurYoga Teacher Training Manual.* Albuquerque: Ayurvedic Press, 2004.

Paramahansa Yogananda. *Cosmic Chants.* Listen, Listen, Listen To My Heart's Song.

Satchidananda Ashram – Yogaville. *Morning and Evening Prayers.* Buckingham, 1998.

RESOURCES

My greatest resources are my compassionate and loving teachers:

For more information about becoming a yoga teacher, an Ayurvedic practitioner, or a yoga therapist or learning more about how these exciting modalities can enhance your life call 303-432-8099 or email: pyamandala@gmail.com or check out the PranaYoga and Ayurveda Mandala website at www.pyamandala.com

Or contact The Ayurvedic Institute PO Box 23445 Albuquerque, New Mexico 87192 505-294-7572 or www.ayurveda.com

To author welcomes correspondence from readers. She may be reached at:
Melissa J Chaney
E-mail: melissajchaney@gmail.com
Website: http://www.melissajchaney.com
And/or tweet with me @melissajchaney

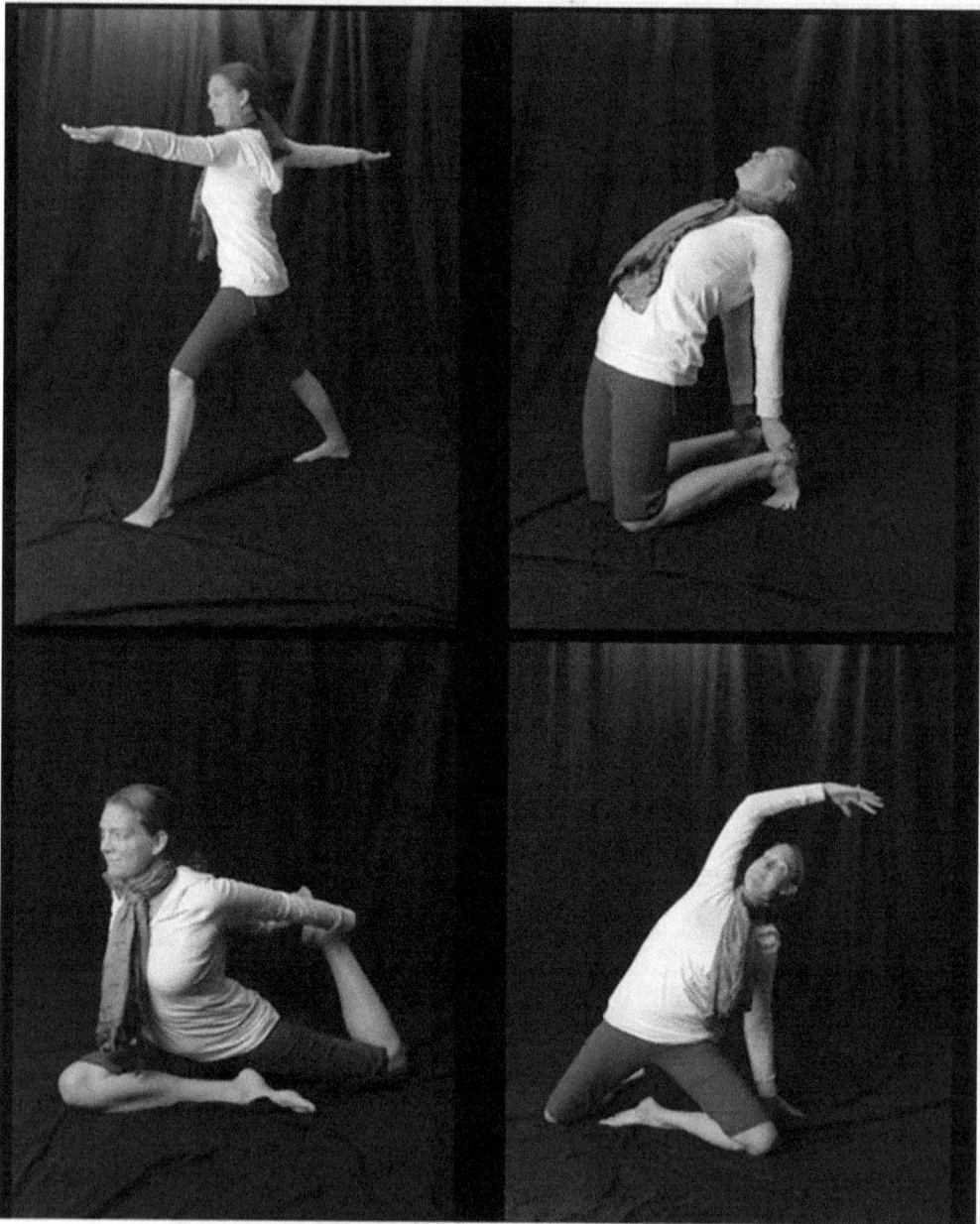

www.ingramcontent.com/pod-product-compliance
Lightning Source LLC
Chambersburg PA
CBHW071329310526
45789CB00017B/2154